Life on the Edge

Life on the Edge
Parenting a Child with ADD/ADHD

David Spohn

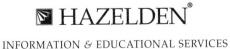

HAZELDEN®

INFORMATION & EDUCATIONAL SERVICES

Hazelden
Center City, Minnesota 55012-0176
1-800-328-0094
1-651-257-1331 (Fax)
www.hazelden.org

02 01 00 99 98   5 4 3 2

Library of Congress Cataloging-in-Publication Data
Spohn, David.
        Life on the edge : parenting a child with ADD/ADHD / David Spohn.
            p.   cm.
        ISBN 1-56838-206-5
        1. Attention-deficit hyperactivity disorder—Popular works. 2. Child rearing.
I. Title.
        RJ506.H9S66 1998
        618.92'8589—dc21
                                                                    98-24858
                                                                       CIP

Cover design, interior design, illustrations by David Spohn
Typesetting by Universal Press, Minneapolis, Minnesota

CONTENTS

Introduction 1

PART 1
Welcome to the Monkey House
"Your Child Has ADD . . . " 7
Your New Vocabulary 9
Your New Friends 11
Mr. Activity and the Shrinking House 13
So, You Thought Your House Was an Investment? 15
Worldly Possessions and the ADD Kid 17
A New Place for the Tools 19

PART 2
Life in the Fast Lane
Looking into Their Eyes 23
The Big Struggle 25
The Ritalin Catch-22 27
Sibling Rivalry 29
Dinnertime 31
Going Out in Public 33

PART 3
School Daze
Classrooms in Motion 37
The Wild Ride 39
Homework 42
Gifted Program or Special Ed? 45
Parents as Advocates 46

PART 4
Surviving and Thriving:
Coping Skills for Parents and Kids
Triscuit Surfing 53
Contracts 56
Care for the Kid, Care for Yourself 59
The ADD Survival Kit 62
Affirmations for the Kid and the Parents 64

PART 5
You Mean He Might Live to Be an Adult?
Teenagers 69
ADD and Chemical Health 71
Hope for the Future 73

HELP! 77
About the Author 81

Introduction

"Life is what happens to you while you're busy making other plans."
—JOHN LENNON

I'll never forget the nightly ritual of rocking our children to sleep. They were active babies, and by their bedtime, my wife and I were just as worn out as they were. We would darken the room, the only lights being the ones that lit the stereo. And holding them firmly, cheek to cheek, we would gently rock and roll them to sleep, swaying to songs from John Lennon and Yoko Ono's *Double Fantasy* album. It worked pretty well, and by the time the music ended, their churning bodies had finally surrendered to sleep.

Years later, we still hear these songs now and then on the radio, and they always take us back to those days. As our kids grew, the words above, from the song "Beautiful Boy," have become even more meaningful.

We look at our newborn babies and imagine the greatest of possibilities. We nourish them with hopes and dreams of a life beyond what we could achieve for ourselves. But each child's life unfolds in its own way. Some seem to walk through life with smooth, easy strides, the wind always at their backs. Some are born with severe challenges that are readily apparent from life's beginning.

For others, childhood gradually becomes more complex, filled with unseen tangles of roots and barbs that make each step increasingly difficult. Life becomes a path of contradictions and catch-22s, marked by failures and frustrations. This is often the life of a child with ADD or ADHD. As parents of these kids, we alternately curse the barbs, soothe the wounds they inflict, and blame ourselves and the child for ending up on such a path. It's not quite what we'd had in mind.

When my wife and I were starting our family, my mother passed along a saying from her mother: "Each baby brings its own bread." At the time, I thought it referred to having the money to simply feed a new child. As a parent of an ADD child, I now see it means much more. Though distractible, driven by impulse, and often burdened with other learning or emotional challenges, many kids with ADD tend not only to be bright, creative thinkers, but often have a surprising ability to fully understand their condition as well. Along with that, of course, they usually have an infinite amount of energy. Just the tools they need!

The most important thing they need now is a circle of support, including properly equipped parents. This proper equipment includes knowledge, energy, patience, and adaptability. Also needed is the willingness to be a disciplinarian and an informed advocate. It's also helpful to be able to laugh in the face of chaos. This is equipment that can be acquired along the way, with a little help and lots of practice. Be assured that help is available, and the practice is daily! By binding these elements together with love, we can guide our children through the maze that is their childhood. This may not be the parenting experience we asked for, but for some of us, it's the one we got. Our kids can and do grow up to be healthy, happy people. And when we filter away all the glitter from those dreams we started with, isn't that all we really wanted anyway?

PART 1

Welcome to the Monkey House

"Your Child Has ADD . . ."

And life as you know it will never be the same

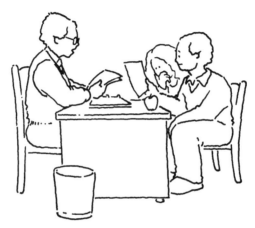

For many of us parents, this diagnosis is one we first hear in the early elementary school years. If our child is hyperactive, we may arrive at this point after hearing such comments from teachers as, "He seems bright enough," "He just can't seem to sit still," "She just can't seem to stay on task," or something to this effect. The added element of hyperactivity may lead to suspicion of ADHD, or attention deficit hyperactivity disorder.

Where hyperactivity isn't an issue, recognizing the presence of ADD—attention deficit disorder—is more difficult, and it may go undetected until much later. Comments about these children might be, "She really doesn't cause any trouble, but . . . ," or "He just doesn't seem interested." Finally, at this point, a psychologist or psychiatrist may sum up an assessment with a diagnosis of ADD or ADHD—terms that I alternate between throughout this book. Either way, the words, "Your child has ADD," are words that change our lives forever.

Some parents react with denial: "There's nothing wrong with *my* child!" Others feel a sense of relief in knowing that, even though their child can spin his head in a 360-degree rotation, he may not necessarily be possessed by demons.

This is a point at which mystery and uncertainty can be replaced by acceptance and resolve. Life as we have known it may never be the same, but at least we now know what we're dealing with. Welcome to Life on the Edge.

Your New Vocabulary

Remember the word-a-day assignments you were given back in grade school? By learning one new word each day, your vocabulary quickly grew by leaps and bounds. Well, now that you have accepted ADD into your life, the lesson continues. New words will be creeping into your vocabulary on a daily basis once again. An accelerated trip through this lesson might go somewhat as follows:

Distraction, impulsivity, and/or **hyperactivity** lead to the inability to stay on task. These may lead to **interventions,** which may eventually lead to an **assessment.** This, in turn, may lead to a diagnosis of **ADD** (attention deficit disorder) or **ADHD** (attention deficit hyperactivity disorder). There may also be associated **learning disabilities** (LD) or **oppositional defiant disorder** (ODD), maybe even **bipolar disorder.** On the medical front, you will learn about **stimulants** and **antidepressants.** The stimulants include **Ritalin, Dexedrine, Desoxyn, Cylert,** and **Adderall.** The antidepressants include **Wellbutrin, Paxil, Tofranil, Nopramin,** and maybe **clonidine** or **lithium.**

At school, your child will have an **IEP** (individualized education plan). You will hear of laws that guarantee **procedural safeguards** at

9

school. Learn about them! **Section 504** and **IDEA** (the Individuals with Disabilities Education Act) are also terms you'll need to understand.

These are only a few of the many terms and acronyms you'll hear when dealing with your child's school. Learn as much as you can in advance so, when dealing with school issues, you can be what is perhaps your most important new word: an **advocate** for your child. And speaking of advocates, one more new term to learn is **CHADD** (Children and Adults with Attention Deficit Disorder). This is a nationwide organization offering information, support, and advocacy for you and your family, no matter where you live. Your community probably has a local CHADD chapter, as well as other helpful advocacy groups. By all means, bring CHADD into your vocabulary and your life.

Clearly, you have a lot to learn, but it can be managed by approaching it **one day at a time,** just as you did in grade school with the word-a-day assignments. Your vocabulary won't be the only thing that improves with the one-day-at-a-time approach. Your whole life will!

Your New Friends

Life with an ADD child will bring new associates into your life as well. You will meet your child's teacher. You'll probably get to know the **school psychologist** and **counselor,** and you may even meet a **caseworker.** You may also get to know the **assistant principal** better than you ever cared to. Perhaps you'll learn to recognize **"tired teachers"**—the ones who would rather not deal with any child who may have special learning needs. This group includes those who should have changed professions years ago, but just never got around to doing it.

You will meet **psychiatrists, psychologists,** and perhaps **neurologists.** You may become acquainted with **social workers** and **mental health counselors, psychiatric nurses,** and **therapists.** You may meet the **police liaison officer,** maybe even the **probation officer.** As a parent, you may become friends with other parents in a **CHADD** support group.

Why all these people? You may have heard the African proverb "It takes an entire village to raise one child." It's never more true than for a child with ADD.

Forget any stigmas you may have previously associated with having to deal with any of the professionals listed above. Whomever you meet, reserve your judgments about how effectively they can help you and your child. These are *all* people who can help, and you will need plenty of help. Seek it out and embrace it, for your child, your family, and yourself.

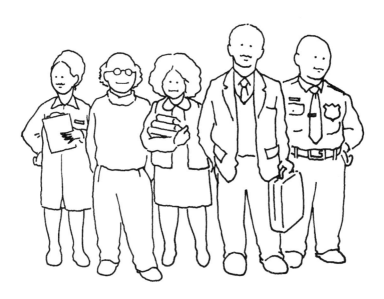

Mr. Activity and the Shrinking House

It seems as if there is not a house built big enough to contain the rambling, usually nonstop energy of an ADHD child. Your child's room probably looks like the epicenter of an 8.6 earthquake, with a trail of debris spilling into the rest of the house. By following this trail, you can trace a random path of activities begun, but abruptly abandoned. And the decibel level accompanying these activities can drive you right through the roof. The key to chaos control is to make some rules and some concessions.

The rules can be built around a couple of simple concepts dealing with respect and boundaries. In our house, the first concept is, "You have the right to swing your arms, but that right ends where my nose begins." The second concept is, "If you don't want it done to you, don't do it to me." You can develop contracts based on these concepts, with rewards and consequences for behavior, but really, they just cover the details. Focusing first on simple concepts improves the chances of having your house rules understood and followed.

Concessions you might consider revolve around your own standards for neatness and your personal space and time. How important is a spotless home with everything in place in relation to conflict and friction with someone who simply cannot grasp your notion of neatness? Flexibility is important here.

One irony of parenting any child is that you always seem to be completely drained of energy at the times you need it most. This is especially true for parents of an ADHD child. Therefore, be sure to build in escape routes ahead of time. When the escalating energy level of your child seems to collide with your need for peace and quiet, try to channel that energy into an activity you can share. If *you* don't have the energy for that, retreat! Give yourself a break when you can, whether it's a weekend getaway or just an evening walk. You give your kids "time-outs," so why not give yourself one too? A rested parent has more patience and perspective than a tired one.

So, You Thought Your House Was an Investment?

Part of the American dream is to own a home of our own. It's a dream that many of us share. This home doesn't need to be a mansion, just a place to raise a family. In addition to seeing it as a shelter from the elements, we envision it to be a shelter from the stresses and cruelties of a sometimes hostile world. Our homes are a tangible expression of who we are, as well. We can often tell a little about the occupants of a home by looking at it. This is certainly true of an ADHD household, in which the house tends to bear evidence of all the slings and arrows of outrageous behavior.

We invest labor, love, and lots of money in this dream, and then we hope for some kind of return. This return often is not what we had in mind: an advanced degree in window replacement with a specialty in spackling or a doctorate in door jamb repair, earned after years of following up from outbursts of ADHD energy, angry or otherwise. During these years of child rearing, it may be best to postpone the investment part of the homeowning dream and live instead for a simpler end. Though it may be hard to believe now, the time we have with our children really is brief. As they grow up, each new step they take is a step away from dependence, away from us. Suddenly they're gone, whether we're ready or not. And when they're gone, chances are the house will still be there. So, I'm frequently reminded of my grandmother's saying, "Dust the living wood first." The rest will still be there, giving us something to do when the house and our lives are a bit more quiet.

Our home is sturdy enough to withstand the challenges of ADHD curiosity and anger. It keeps the rain and snow out, the warmth and love in. That's good enough for now.

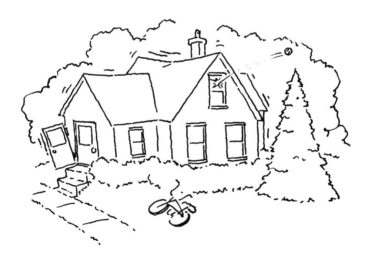

Worldly Possessions and the ADD Kid

Pick one or the other

In our house, you notice the little things. Maybe it's the picture frames whose bottom corners are all smashed. The glass in those corners is cracked too. You see, if you dribble a basketball on the walls long and hard enough, the pictures will eventually leap right off and land on the floor pretty much the same way each time.

Maybe you notice the holes drilled into the furniture, or you find the telephone completely disassembled when you go to make a call. You may find different destruction to a different degree in each house, but it's all the aftermath of a mind racing so quickly that the hands must work furiously to keep up with all the impulses.

Prized possessions, family heirlooms, furniture, even the bathroom fixtures can almost spontaneously turn into debris in the wake of ADD energy. The important thing to remember is that just about all of these objects, no matter what their description or price tag, probably have one major thing in common: They're replaceable, and your child isn't.

Of course, we don't *really* need to pick one or the other. Even ADD kids need to learn to live in the material world. In this world there are some rules, and there will be some losses. This is another instance where a combination of discipline and accommodations is needed. Yes, the house rules include a restriction on bouncing a basketball on the walls. But at the same time, Plexiglas can be the replacement material of choice when the pictures hit the floor. We all like tables to eat at and furniture to sit on, but how important is it to have the finest of these things at this time in our lives?

And the truly prized possessions can be kept in a safe place—with the understanding, of course, that almost anywhere in the house may still be considered in harm's way. If you work at this issue from both ends, it's possible to teach responsible behavior, cut material losses, and eliminate a few points of conflict.

A New Place for the Tools

All over the yard

Does this sound familiar? You need to repair something around the house, so you go to your toolbox to get your screwdriver and wrench. However, your toolbox is open, and the tools you need are nowhere to be found. After a brief, exasperating search and a fruitless interrogation of the usual suspect(s), you determine that the chore must be left for another time. Several days later, while you're mowing the lawn, a jarring *clunk* stops the lawnmower dead in its tracks. Upon inspection of the underside of the lawnmower, you observe a sizable gouge in the blade. And there on the ground, a bit rustier than when you last saw it, is your wrench. At least you got it back this time. Other tools have vanished, never to be seen again.

The ADHD mind is an active one, always looking for something to take apart, and sometimes even put back together again. This requires tools or other belongings we'd probably rather not have tampered with. At our house, rules and boundaries regarding worldly possessions such as the toolbox have been a frequent issue. Since ADHD kids often are kinesthetic learners, the process of learning just about anything is a hands-on experience. Thus, each learning experience, at least in our

19

house, can often be traced by following the trail of tools, spare parts, and debris left around the house or yard. After a great deal of frustration, we solved this by giving our child a toolbox of his own. It's not necessarily a perfect solution, but the goal here is not to achieve perfection.

The guiding principle is to find successes, no matter how small, wherever they can be found. Tools will still turn up half-buried in the yard, but an extra set of tools that my child can call his own will also improve my chances of finding a wrench when I really need one. You, as well, may find that the child who cannot seem to create order in any area of his life, may be able to succeed in keeping a perfectly organized toolbox of his own.

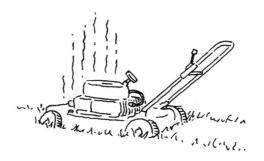

PART 2

Life in the Fast Lane

Looking into Their Eyes

"Is anybody in there?"

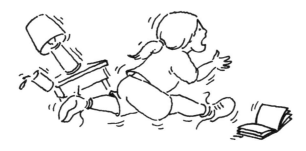

Your child's voice gets loud and shrill; her cheeks turn bright red. Her activity level rapidly escalates to critical mass. She seems oblivious to requests to slow down, and your patience is about to give in to anger. You grab hold of the child—a frenzied, turbulent, overheated body in motion. You look into her eyes to rivet your command for attention, but there seems to be no one there. The eyes you look into are glazed and stare right back through you. After an endless moment of being held in place, calm returns to your child and her eyes are able to focus, meeting your own. If you have succeeded in keeping your own cool, you try to guide the child into a less frantic mode. This is a hallmark moment recognized by any parent with an ADHD child.

Later, when these kids can better verbalize their feelings, they express their struggle to control their minds and bodies: "I just don't know why I did that." "I just want to be normal." But that look in their eyes is very telling. Their message is that this chaos is not the work of the devil. This is not a child trying to drive you insane. This is a child unable to control her actions, who, if she could, would love nothing more than to sit and read or play like any other child. Recognizing this expression can help us look past the body that is out of control, past the mind that can't focus to the heart that has the same desire as any other child's: to grow and be happy. Recognizing this expression can lead us past anger and frustration to compassion.

Recognizing this expression is the foundation for all the therapy, parenting skills, and teaching strategies that will be needed to help this child grow. The child may be healthy, strong, and as bright as can be. But the child is also like a race car roaring on all cylinders, with a driver looking at the road through a kaleidoscope. Yes, these kids must learn to become accountable for and control their behavior. But to do so, they must have help learning to cope with the disability that stands in their way. And, through thick and thin, this help must always be grounded in compassion.

The Big Struggle

Sometimes, things just get out of hand. When the child escalates to that critical mass stage, just about anything can happen. The characteristics of escalated ADHD behavior are like those of a tornado: loud, dangerous, and able to suck everyone and everything in its path into its vortex. Faced with the shrill voice, the bright red cheeks, and those glazed eyes, how loud and forcefully must you express yourself to be heard? It's so easy to be drawn into the fury. The ADHD personality loves company and would like nothing better than to draw you into the storm.

This is the Big Struggle—a term coined by Edward Hallowell in *Driven to Distraction*—and it's not pretty. Every parent of an ADHD child knows what this is, and it is here that we as parents must learn to keep control of our emotions. This is *much* easier said than done. Yes, it is frustrating to try to manage a child who will not listen, obey, or simply control himself. It's frustrating to have a child's wildly impulsive behavior take over a family meal, activity, or quiet time. This frustration and anger can easily get the best of us, making us part of the problem instead of the solution. And once you've been drawn into the Big Struggle, what do you think your chances are of out-ADHDing the ADHD child?

Time out! If your kid won't take one, then *you* must, even if it means you don't get the last word. If you can't reach a loud and raging child with a soft and calm voice, it may be better to just get out of the way. In terms of personal chemistry, the effect of using confrontation to control ADHD behavior is the rough equivalent of applying gasoline to fire.

Ask for help from your partner, if possible. Also, learn to look for your child's HALT signs—he may really be *hungry, angry, lonely,* or *tired.* Check out these possibilities first, find out what your child is really trying to ask for, and then approach the behavior problem. Remember, tornadoes are loud, violent, and frightening, but they usually pass quickly.

Learning to avoid the Big Struggle is an art. It requires constant vigilance over our emotions. It requires an ability to anticipate conditions that could lead to troublesome situations. It requires that parents look out for each other as well as for their child, and help each other out when one or the other is vulnerable (learn to look for your own HALT signs as well). It's enough having one person in the family escalating out of control. Do you really want two?

The Ritalin Catch-22
"Oops, I forgot to take it"

Of *course* she forgot to take her medication! If she could remember to take it, she probably wouldn't need it in the first place. It's just another of the cruel ironies that comes with the ADD experience. About the only thing that can really top this is trying to convince the 35 to 65 percent of ADD kids who are also diagnosed with ODD (oppositional defiant disorder) that they need the medication at all. What it frequently adds up to for parents is a case of EDD (emotionally drained and depressed).

There really isn't a perfect solution. As we've discovered before, however, some imperfect ones will do. For better or for worse, in many cases, medication is an important part of the effective treatment of ADD. And for better or for worse, the child must bear at least part of the responsibility for the treatment. As parents, we can create many mechanisms to see that the child remembers to take it. We can make lists and notes and leave them in strategic places. We can buy inexpensive plastic weekly medication management kits for organizing and more expensive electronic organizers for remembering. Both of these are perfect toys for hyperactive fingers. Whatever works, for however long, however cumbersome it seems, is worth a try. Today, do what works for today. Tomorrow, do what works for tomorrow. Next week, next month . . .

At any rate, we can't lose sight of the fact that medication isn't the cure-all. At best, it represents one portion of a program that should also include education, therapeutic help, and coping skills for the child and the family, as well as behavioral management and ongoing work with the school. If we only concentrate on the medication, it's not long before we're dealing with a child who feels she's being drugged just to be kept quiet. Remember the big picture, and expect to see the pill still sitting on the breakfast table after the school bus pulls away. Just try again tomorrow.

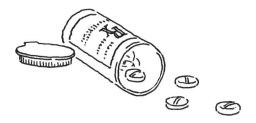

Sibling Rivalry
Blood brothers and bloodshed

There may be no bond as powerful as brotherhood. And, at any given time, there may be no more powerful hold than that of a child's hands around his brother's throat. Growing up with siblings prepares us for a social world. We learn how to share, how to negotiate, and yes, we learn how to fight. Above all, though, we learn about unconditional love. Most brothers and sisters consider their siblings both a blessing and a curse, depending upon the moment. A child with an ADHD sibling will naturally see the curse, and must be shown how to see the blessings.

It can be hard to see blessings when the effects of a sibling's ADHD behavior spill over into the lives of everyone in the family. They're hard to see when there seems to be no escape from a sibling who constantly invades your space; takes, loses, or destroys your things; embarrasses you in front of your friends; and pushes your parents to the edge of a rage that always seems to come out at you. It's hard to see blessings when the ADHD child in the family gets so much attention and so much accommodation. How can you be expected to deal with your brother's ADHD when you're struggling to figure out your own life?

For the ADHD child, on the other hand, the struggle is in seeing a sibling for whom everything seems so easy and so right, who always earns praise and privileges, who enjoys friendships and success. How do you get along with someone against whom you never seem to measure up?

This is a challenge for the whole family. We, as parents, must keep our eyes on the prize for our kids. We may not be able to treat them the same, but we must treat them fairly. We must be careful to understand each of their different needs, remembering also to grease the wheels that don't squeak. We must get a firm grasp on the good times our children have together and savor them. These times will fuel our hope for the future.

The blessings are there, though they might only be realized later in life. The child living with an ADHD sibling will develop patience and a greater understanding of people's differences. The ADHD child will receive support and a good example. None of these blessings will seem apparent or meaningful now, but they can be the foundation for a lifelong relationship of unconditional love, long after Mom and Dad are around to keep the peace.

Dinnertime

Family tradition meets the aerobic eater

We'd like to pass on to our children the customs we grew up with. One of the most cherished of these customs is a nice, quiet sit-down dinner. This is often the only time all day when the entire family can come together and enjoy each other's company. In an ADD household, however, this doesn't always work out as planned.

By now, it has become evident that doing anything that requires sitting for any amount of time can be challenging for a kid with ADD. While most family members can sit, eat, and share the experiences of their day, the aerobic eater is often more at home performing. Like any performer, this one needs to project with volume, gesture dramatically, and generally do whatever it takes to command the attention of the audience. Thus, this situation has definite potential for conflict. But beyond the projectiles of flying food, the teetering glasses of milk, and our own churning stomachs, what we really have is a kid telling us about his day.

After all, a day in the life of an ADD child is probably quite a bit more eventful and adventuresome than most people's day. Yes, we want to eat a peaceful meal together, and we also want to teach proper table

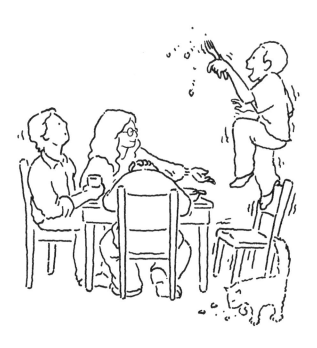

manners, as we learned them. But sometimes, for the sake of peace, harmony, and proper digestion for the entire family, tradition can make room for one who has just as much to tell, but who has a different way of answering the question, "So, how was your day?"

Going Out in Public
"Yes, this is my kid. So what?"

Yes, there's nothing quite like a loud, public display of acting out by your child to make you feel completely incompetent and dysfunctional. If such displays weren't enough to cope with at home, they are even worse when they occur in a busy grocery store, mall, or at a school or social function. The turned heads and disapproving stares can add to the frustration you're already feeling. ADD kids don't have trained behavioral guide dogs. They don't have large ID bracelets that announce to the world that they have an attention deficit disorder that may include other psychological and/or learning problems. To the rest of the world, they just look like spoiled, out-of-control kids. And you, of course, look like a helpless, ineffective parent.

Here's a suggestion in two parts: The first involves separating the child's behavior from your own. Who's acting out, anyway? Chances are it's your child, not you. Don't be embarrassed by behavior that isn't yours. Second, although people may pass judgment on you as a parent by what they see, who needs to impress such judgmental people anyway? Unless the behavior is truly causing someone harm, it's simply none of their business. They know nothing about what you're dealing with as a parent, and you owe them no explanation. Ignore the stares as best you can and go about doing what you need to do. In time, no matter how shy or polite you are, you can perfect a disparaging glare that is strong enough to return a stranger's attention to his or her own affairs.

Doing and being what's expected of you and keeping up appearances of normalcy can be a huge burden. This is especially true when life presents you with what you didn't expect and when normal is a concept that rarely applies to your life. Sometimes, it's just best to free yourself and simply not give a damn about what other people think. This way, you can stay focused on what really matters and what really commands your attention: teaching your child, as best you can, how to behave in a social world.

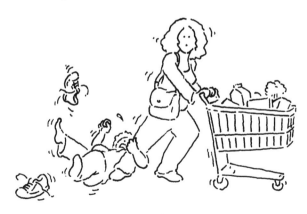

PART 3

School Daze

Classrooms in Motion

The kinesthetic learner

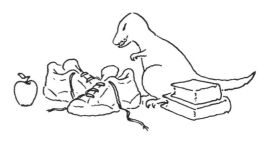

The elementary school years pass so quickly, they are often just a blur. For a parent with an ADD child, they are even blurrier. Often, second or third grade is the period in which children suspected of having attention deficits are first identified. That was our experience. As a parent, you may receive your first clue when your child brings home a report card with grades that aren't as good as you'd hoped or when you receive frequent calls from the teacher. It may be a conference where the teacher looks tired and exasperated or struggles to find positive things to say about your child.

Whatever the signs are, follow them. In the elementary years, parents can more easily be in touch with what happens at school. If you suspect or confirm that your child has ADD or ADHD, get involved. It can make the difference between your child's waging a daily war or having a teacher who understands and is willing to modify the classroom setting, strategies, and expectations to fit your child's needs.

Our son's best year in grade school was the year he had a teacher who really recognized what it meant to be ADHD. They made a deal. Our son could go anywhere in the classroom at any time and could explore any of the many activities that were set up. In turn, he could not disrupt anyone, and he needed to be able to reasonably answer questions and participate verbally when called upon. As long as those conditions were met, he had complete freedom in the room. This teacher understood that many ADHD kids are kinesthetic learners. They learn by doing. They simply need to be active to absorb information. They concentrate on many things at once, although, as indicated by the trail of chaos left behind, they seem unable to concentrate at all. In this case it worked—perhaps because the teacher in this case seemed to have ADHD himself.

Teachers like this open up greater opportunities for ADD kids. Instead of taking written tests and writing reports, perhaps a child can make models of history subjects, act out math problems, and dress up as literary characters. For others who may be auditory learners, the solution may be as simple as taking tests orally. There are many different learning styles, and no one style should be valued over another. At this point, it is up to us to make sure our children have a classroom situation they can succeed in.

The Wild Ride

Life on the school bus

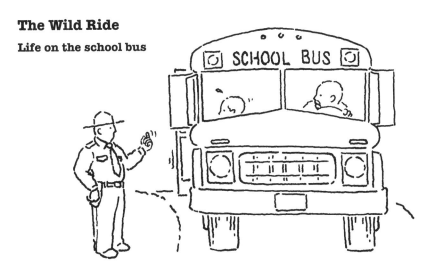

I can laugh at this event now, but it wasn't so funny at the time. We got this story from the principal, who described the incident according to the state trooper's report. Our son, then a fourth-grader, had climbed out the window of a moving school bus far enough to reach out onto the roof, pack a perfect snowball, and let it fly. Right on target, he hit an oncoming car (which happened to be the trooper) square in the center of its windshield. At 55 miles per hour, the impressiveness of this feat was diminished somewhat by the poor judgment involved.

There were many other school bus incidents, but this is the one that stands out. The school bus was a constant concern, and our son was regularly suspended from riding it. The ride in the morning wasn't a problem, just the afternoon ride home. Looking back, the whole situation was as predictable as the setting sun. Take a kid with boundless energy and impulsive tendencies, then constrain that energy for about six hours in a school situation that is at best frustrating. At the end of the day, put him into a completely unstructured setting with several dozen other kids who are also ready to bust loose. Then make sure that the only adult present—the driver—is facing the direction opposite the children and engaged in an activity that requires complete attention: driving.

Sound like a perfect recipe for chaos? For the child with ADHD, it would defy logic to be anything other than completely out of control. So, why set the situation up if it can be avoided? A child assessed as having ADHD is just as eligible as anyone else for transportation services to and from school, but it doesn't have to be the regular school bus. If the school bus is a constant problem, consider the smaller form of transportation used for kids with special needs. The number of kids on this type of bus is much smaller, and the atmosphere on board is much more conducive to everyone's safety. The Individuals with Disabilities Education Act

(IDEA) provides for such service as part of the guaranteed right to a free public education for all children. An ADHD diagnosis can make a child eligible for special transportation if that's what is needed.

Parents with kids who have ADHD have many challenges to deal with. There's no sense struggling with one that can simply be eliminated by arranging for another means of transportation. Some kids will respond really well and, in fact, be a positive presence for some of the needier riders. Others might resist, feeling stigmatized. Fine. Then you may have room to negotiate the issue of bus behavior and consequences.

Homework

Just whose is it anyway?

Ever worry about all that stuff you missed or just didn't understand in school? Well, lucky for you, if you're the parent of an ADD child, you'll get to catch up on all of it the second time around. Yes, all it will take is following the trail of missed and misplaced assignments, as well as nightly homework wars, to bring you up to speed. When they handed our son his certificate at his grade school graduation, part of me wanted to jump up and yell out, "Hey, wait a minute, that's mine!"

Homework is a huge challenge for parents because it's a huge challenge for any kid with ADD. From the organizational aspect of remembering to bring the right material home to the task of dealing with written assignments, reading, and math, this challenge is full of potential for conflict. The average half-hour assignment can easily become an all-out, all-evening ordeal. It's amazing how a child can spend three hours struggling through evasive maneuvers to avoid having to do an assignment that could be completed in fifteen minutes. It's exhausting and frustrating for everyone involved. But we have learned some things along the way.

As with so many of these issues, the solutions seem to be small

42

adjustments in several areas. First, talk to the teacher. Arrange for a check-in at the end of the day to make sure the right material finds its way home. Just be aware that even this will not eliminate the occasional trip back to school to pick up what was forgotten. Also, instead of having your child complete a sheet of twenty math problems, suggest that your child do every other one, to show that the comprehension is there. This is a common strategy with ADD kids, as the act of writing out the problem and keeping the paper in one piece is a challenge in itself. If possible, substitute learning activities, models, costumes, whatever, for the dreaded worksheets. Then, find ways to make the time spent on homework as enjoyable as possible.

You'll find little things that work if you look hard enough. Aim for that elusive space where you can facilitate without overstepping your bounds. Expect imperfection and reward effort. In the end, it is your child's homework, not yours or mine.

And what about that conventional wisdom that says children must have a quiet place in their room set aside for study? You may want to reconsider that. For our son, the best place for homework was right under our noses, at the kitchen table, either right before or right after supper. Quiet? Nope. A space reserved for homework? Nope. Our kitchen is the busiest room in the house. But we found we could retrieve and redirect wandering attention more quickly if we were closer at hand. Kinesthetic learners don't necessarily need quiet in order to absorb information. And as long as the work gets done, who cares about a little ketchup or jelly on the paper?

Finally, there's the issue of getting homework turned in. As parents, try as you may, you pretty much have to let go of that one. So my advice here is for the teacher: Look in that wadded-up pile at the bottom of his locker. It's probably there.

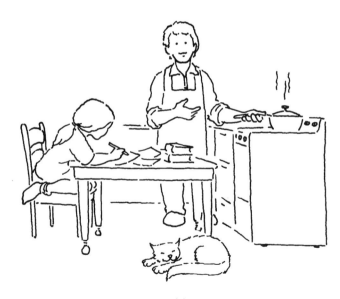

Gifted Program or Special Ed?

This should have been one of our first clues: Deluged by all the paper churned out by the school system, I remember being puzzled when a report came home stating that our son—then in early elementary school—was identified as a candidate for the high potential program; then another came that identified him as a student in need of remedial support in reading and math.

Now, with the benefit of a few years of perspective, it makes more sense. Here was a kid with a lively imagination, great curiosity, boundless energy, and a thousand interests. At the same time, this was a kid for whom a fill-in-the-circle test form presented the opportunity to create a dot-to-dot picture. The last thing he would think of doing would be to fill in the circle appropriate to the answer of some (allegedly) corresponding question. What could those circles possibly have to do with math, science, history, or literature?

In a way, this was a glimpse into the future. It was a hint of the disconnect that can often occur between kids with ADD and the school system into which they struggle to fit. Beware of clues that pop up like this. They're a call to action.

Parents as Advocates

Educating the educators

And sooner rather than later, the action comes! The older our kids get, the more complicated it becomes to stay abreast of their school lives. In middle school or junior high, our kids have four, five, six, or more teachers to deal with instead of just one. Classes are set up to accommodate kids who can sit at a desk all day, listen to a teacher's lecture, take notes, fill out worksheets, jot down homework assignments in a notebook, remember to take that notebook home along with the necessary materials, do the work, and remember to bring it in and return it the next day. Most tests consist of multiple-choice problems, fill-in-the-blank statements, or essays. Children are judged either a success or failure based on their ability to perform well in these tasks. Even the passing times in the halls between classes challenge their self-control. The ADD child, no matter how bright or enthusiastic, can find this setting to be very difficult.

Inability to succeed in this type of environment can lead to acting out, discipline problems, and labels such as EBD (emotionally behaviorally disturbed). Sometimes the child may be bored with an educational structure he cannot relate to. Or, the acting out may simply be the release of pent-up energy. This energy must be vented somehow, because the teaching style cannot harness it. It's frustrating to be cast into a system that does not work for you and even punishes you for your natural learning style.

Teacher conferences can be intimidating, even shaming, when your child has problems in school. Some teachers and administrators will view your child's problems as your failure as a parent. This naturally raises the emotional stakes, but try to withhold judgment about your child's performance or actions (or your own parental ability) until you have had time to consider the whole picture.

A seventh-grade geography teacher once told us that our son seemed totally lost and disinterested, that he was a complete disruption, and that the class was "so much better when he wasn't there." Just days later, this same boy used a long car ride to his basketball game to happily share what he had learned in school about latitude and longitude, and relative latitudinal and longitudinal relationships of places around the world in great depth. He knew how it all worked, but he was failing the class. I wondered who was really lost and disinterested, the child or the teacher and the system he was part of.

Schools have limited resources available to accommodate those whose learning style requires a different type of environment. As with children with learning disabilities, public schools are legally required to provide accommodations for children assessed as having ADD. Here is where you need to be prepared. If you do not have an assessment, get one done. This can be done by the school or you can have one done on your own, usually with a referral from your family doctor or the school. Whether you like the idea of an ADD or ADHD label being placed on your child doesn't matter. This may be the key to help in school.

Since ADD is included in the Individuals with Disabilities Education Act (IDEA), these children are entitled by law to a variety of accommodations, more numerous than can be mentioned here. They are entitled to an Individual Education Plan (IEP) developed to fit their needs. Parents are entitled to participate in developing this plan. IDEA also places limits on disciplinary action that can be taken when problems arise. Your child is entitled to whatever it takes to make a free public education available. It's the law. But it is up to you to make sure that the proper services are provided and that your child's rights are protected. Most school administrators are helpful and knowledgeable in this area, but others are too busy, too tired, not aware, or would rather not have their lives complicated with such issues.

Learn about IDEA and learn about how to create a good IEP. Your school should have literature available explaining these protections. Just ask them. Whether it's providing an extra set of books to keep at home for the child who cannot remember to bring them from school; abbreviated assignments; untimed, supervised, or even oral tests; a classroom aide; or even a shortened school day, there is much that can be done. But it will take your getting involved. Find the teachers or administrators who care the most and enlist their help. Then, help them. Work with them and show them your appreciation. If you're not satisfied with the school's efforts, get help from the outside. There are advocacy groups who can help you (some of them are listed at the end of this book).

The educational system presents a maze for anyone with special needs. Your child will need your help negotiating this system. Arm yourself with energy, information, and willingness to be an advocate.

And here's a thought to tuck away for safekeeping: Your child's success or failure in school isn't necessarily a measure of her success or failure in adult life.

PART 4

Surviving and Thriving:
Coping Skills for Parents and Kids

Triscuit Surfing

Special talents: find them, nurture them

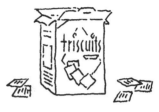

All it took was to move into a house with a few electrical peculiarities to discover the electrician in our son. As I struggled with a fairly simple repair job, he watched, eager to help. Then he ventured, "Why don't you let me give that a try?" Before I knew it, I was the one watching, occasionally fetching tools or materials. Then the job was done. It reminded me of an incident several years before, when, as a youngster, he came outside to watch me change the oil in the car. He amazed me by looking under the hood for the first time and clearly explaining what all those parts to the engine were and how they made the car run. My son can simply look at something, and, as I watch his eyes, I can see how quickly he understands how it works.

For ADD children who so often find that their efforts come up short, whether in school or in their relationships, finding success is critical to their self-esteem. School experiences can often damage these kids' views of themselves. Our son failed science miserably at school, but he knows all about electricity and has a keen understanding of the natural world of animals, food chains, and the environment. He thinks he's dumb, while I marvel at his ability to learn quickly and in his own way. Needless to say, this makes it important to find and acknowledge the things that your child is interested in and does well at. When these talents reveal themselves, pounce on them. Surround the child with whatever materials you can muster to support that interest. Most important, surround him with encouragement.

Don't discount talents that may seem trivial or useless. Let me give an example: One day I was driving home with my son, and we were both tired, hungry, and crabby. He was devouring a box of Triscuits. Once he filled up on them, the remaining crackers in the box took on a purpose their inventors never could have dreamed of. My son rolled down the window as we cruised down the highway and let the wind current play his hand like the wing of an airplane. Before long, I looked over to see his hand spread out, his long fingers piercing the wind. He was balancing a Triscuit vertically against his index fingertip, with only the force of the wind keeping it from flying away. At first I warned him about the fine for littering, then about the

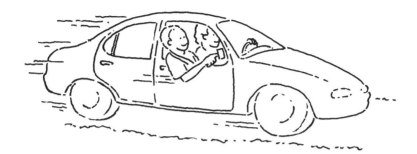

dangers of waving your limbs out a car window. But after he had his second and third finger each tipped with a Triscuit, I couldn't help myself. "That's great!" I said. "See if you can get one up on each finger." By the time we turned off the highway and cruised down our road, he was beaming, five Triscuits to the wind. We came in the house laughing and tried (not very successfully) to explain the invention of a new sport to the rest of our family. Triscuit surfing, it was dubbed.

A number of times since then we've been in the car together, just as tired, hungry, and crabby. And all it's taken to crack the mood has been a brief round of Triscuit surfing. I'm not very good at this myself, but I'm delighted that my son discovered his own form of relaxation therapy. I'm not sure which is the greater accomplishment, the ability to Triscuit surf or simply the ability to discover such a unique way to unwind.

Contracts
The carrot and the stick

The impulsive ADHD mind can go full tilt toward a different direction or interest every day, with the associated wants and needs quickly becoming absolute demands. One day the child wants to get into skateboarding—NOW!—and must have the board, the right shoes, a cool shirt, the whole works. The next day, it's the unquenchable thirst for a dirt bike and, of course, the helmet, the suit, the tools, and everything else associated with it. Then it's on to something else. Interests spring up suddenly and spontaneously, usually skipping the casual-interest phase and proceeding immediately to full-blown passion. These interests never seem to be of the more mundane type: competitive dishwashing, power bed making, and so on. And with the exception of Triscuit surfing, they also never seem to be cheap.

Trying to keep up with this can be dizzying. Of course, you don't want to be the one to dampen unexplored interests (well, at least not most of the time). But how do you slow down the thinking enough to harness some of that energy to help around the house? Or to separate the passing fancies from potential lifelong passions?

One of the most helpful concepts we've come upon is the contract. It's as basic and as American as apple pie. A written document with the child's signature on it is a visible, tangible object capable of lengthening the shortest of attention spans. This can open the door to achieving longer-term goals than would otherwise be possible. The goal can be to earn something special or it can simply be a way of getting the homework done. Maybe the goal is to develop a routine of regular household chores in exchange for a weekly allowance. Making a contract presents the child with the chance to earn what she wants. She also learns negotiating skills, and you get to help cultivate responsible behavior. You can find models to use or you can just make up your own; whatever works. Contracts, proposed with all the terms clearly spelled out, also force the child to think about just how badly she wants what she wants.

Our budding basketball star felt in his heart that in order to achieve his full athletic potential, he had to have the most expensive shoes ever known to the sport. I, however, remembered playing pretty well as a kid in the same kind of shoes that everyone else wore, including the pros, and that cost about twenty bucks. We were at an impasse. But as the season drew nearer and the sky began to threaten snow, he came up with a deal I couldn't refuse: his gazillion-dollar basketball shoes in return for snow removal service for the entire winter—a Minnesota winter, no less—whether it snowed once all year or dumped a foot a day. A deal was quickly struck.

We put the agreement on paper, with a signed copy for each of us. And the kid who could rarely follow through with what he promised never once wavered in his commitment. That year we had near-record snowfall. Halfway through the winter, he had cleared so much snow that I felt guilty about how little those shoes had cost me compared with the price he was paying. We finished the winter sharing the responsibility, and he enjoyed his basketball season in high style. He was proud of his shoes, and he was proud that he had worked hard to earn them. He was also proud that he had been able to start something, stick with it over a long period of time, and finally see it through. And it was all down in black and white. Now he comes to us not so often with demands, but with proposals. Some are doable, some are not. But that's life, isn't it?

Care for the Kid, Care for Yourself

Mr. Magic Fingers' relaxation therapy

The energy created in any ADD house has a natural by-product: tension and stress for everyone. It's important to know how to deal with it and defuse it. Relaxation techniques are necessary to help ADHD kids (and adults as well) learn to calm down. Simple breathing techniques and massage are a couple that work well.

Deep breathing is fairly simple for anyone to learn and is helpful because it can be done just about anywhere, anytime, all by yourself. The results are immediate, and they promote calm, clear thinking. It's kind of like taking a time-out to reboot. Massage works well because kinesthetic people—which describes many ADD people, and especially many ADHD people—respond well to human touch. You don't even need to be a professional massage therapist. In our family Mom does happen to be a certified massage therapist, but simply being able to give a nice back, shoulder, or neck rub can work wonders.

There are other fascinating techniques used in therapeutic settings, including one in which the relaxee is rolled up in a blanket to calm down. The theory is that, although ADHD people may seem insensitive, they are the opposite. They actually are hypersensitive, reacting and responding to everything at once. Wrapping up in a blanket seems to insulate the body from all those wild stimuli, allowing the person to calm down. When I first heard of this at a workshop, I was immediately struck by how self-aware my son was. He has always loved to roll himself up in a blanket. And though his room is generally a picture of chaos, the one recognizable area of order is where he sleeps. I wouldn't call it neat, but it usually resembles a cocoon. In his own way, he's always been looking for a way to calm himself down.

He's always seeking human touch as well, whether looking for a massage for sore muscles or just cuddling up with Mom or Dad on the couch. When he was a baby, we were amazed at how he would instinctively grab hold of and rub his earlobes to stop himself from crying or to wind down. In later years, even when he's been at his angriest, it takes just minutes before he wants to cuddle up and be held, massaged, or just touched. Things soon calm down.

On the flip side, Mr. Kinesthetic is amazingly sensitive with his own hands. He's a master at giving massages himself, and nobody needs one more than Mom or Dad. It seems to be the same instinctual knowledge he showed under the hood of the car: knowledge that just seems to be absorbed right up through his fingertips. Even at a young age, he was able to find exactly what part of my shoulders was knotted up and relieve the pressure. This sensitive touch is clearly the upside of being hypersensitive, and it should definitely be cultivated.

Learn all you can about relaxation therapy. Put what you learn into daily practice, on your child and especially on yourself. You'll have another tool available for helping your child, and you may even get a great back rub out of it.

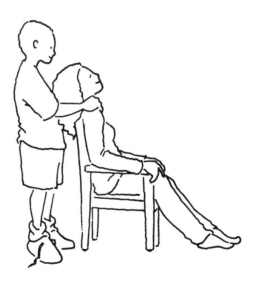

The ADD Survival Kit
The toolbox for getting through the day

You don't have to have ADD to feel organizationally challenged these days. Today's accelerated world is increasingly full of products and gadgets to keep us going where we need to be going. This is good news when looking for little things that can help a person cope with ADD. A parent can find a wide range of devices to help with this, from simple to complex. Pads of stick-on notes to write reminders on and plastic dispensers to help with medication management are simple, inexpensive aids. Alarm watches, calculators, pagers, electronic personal organizers, and calendars are some of the more complex devices available. Any of them can be helpful.

Of course, as always, no solution is perfect. But start with the simple approach: Make lists! This makes sense for anyone, but it can be a great habit for anyone with ADD. Stick-on notes are great because they can be stuck just about anywhere. You can stick one right to your child's forehead if you want—but then she has to remember to read it. Some of the more expensive personal organizers can remind a child to take medication or remember where to be at a given time. But before you invest in one of these, consider how often homework, books, or even shoes tend to disappear at school or on the bus. Pick and choose. Experiment.

The more you think about the problems of forgetfulness and disorganization, the more solutions you'll come up with on your own. Some may even show up unsolicited. One of the best devices we have came in the mail courtesy of a local real estate agent—the best junk mail we ever got. It's a large refrigerator magnet with a wipeable vinyl notepad and pen attached. I've long since tired of looking at that agent's mug shot and logo, but what a small price for such a great tool. It's big enough to display several reminders at once in bold letters and can be wiped clean with a damp cloth. Even the real estate agent's mantra provided good advice: "Location, location, location!" In a household containing an ADHD teenager, could there be a better place than the door to the refrigerator?

Life on the Edge, remember, is a day-to-day experience. Find what works and use it until it doesn't work anymore. Then find something else. It might feel like a life held together with duct tape, but if that's so, just keep plenty of duct tape in your survival kit.

Affirmations for the Kid and the Parents

Our ADD kids are pounded so regularly with messages that point out their shortcomings, it's important to counter them with messages of encouragement.

That message board on the refrigerator is a good place to start. Any kind of positive thought that is short enough to be repeated during breakfast and remembered through the trials of a school day will work. We have found them in all kinds of sources: daily meditation books, daily calendars, cartoon strips, even television commercials. Make some up. We all need to be reminded of our virtues and value, so find some for yourself too.

Here are a few to start with. Try these, and then go find some for yourself!

FOR THE KID

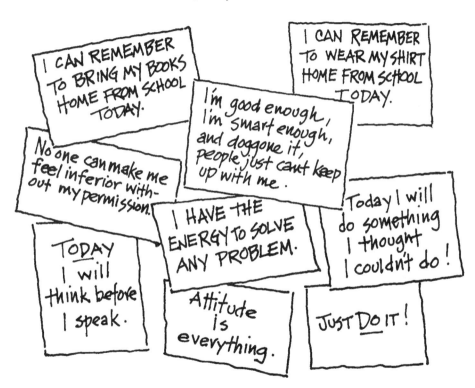

FOR YOURSELF

A journey of a thousand miles begins with a single step.
LAO-TZU

Most folks are about as happy as they make up their minds to be.
ABRAHAM LINCOLN

A mother's heart is a child's school room.
HENRY WARD BEECHER

Muddy water, let stand, becomes clear.
LAO-TZU

PATIENCE is a virtue that carries a lot of wait.

It's not the weight of the burden that matters as much as the manner in which it's carried.

TODAY
I will look past the shortcomings to find the hidden talents.

The essence of being human is that one does not seek perfection.
GEORGE ORWELL

I will face the challenges of this day with compassion and acceptance.

66

PART 5

You Mean He Might Live to Be an Adult?

Teenagers

Boundless energy versus reckless abandon

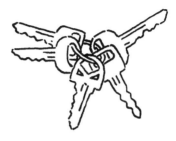

The energy level of people with ADHD can wither anyone around them. The irony is that most of us probably envy such energy. It's a double-edged sword. We think that if we had that much energy, there'd be no limit to what we could accomplish. Yet, this same quality, combined with ADD, can have chaotic, even destructive results. The difference is having the ability to slow down, take stock, and think things out. It comes down to reasoning and decision-making skills.

It seems, however, that reasoning and decision-making skills are words rarely used in the same sentence as the word "teenager." Life is complicated enough for any teenager. When you throw ADD into the mix of puberty, learning to drive, increased independence, and all the other passages into adulthood, we're talking about a real adventure!

Behaviors that we used to chuckle over a few years ago become more serious. Now the ability or inability to interact socially means the difference between having friends and being isolated. Or it means the difference between the type of friends chosen. Decision-making skills and control over impulsive behavior can be life-and-death issues when car keys or alcohol and other drugs are involved.

Are you ready to turn your car over to the same kid who can barely complete a phone call without completely disassembling the telephone? Teenage drivers in general are the highest risk of any age group, and their insurance premiums reflect this. Statistics also show that drivers with ADD tend to have more accidents than others. They also get four times as many tickets. So add all this together, and be prepared. Maybe driving privileges are something to be introduced more gradually with ADD kids. Maybe a contract tied to other areas of home and school life will help. And maybe a bigger, slower car is in order.

Our kids become teenagers whether we're ready or not. The better prepared we are, the smoother the transition for all of us. Buckle up and enjoy the ride!

ADD and Chemical Health

How can you tell *me* not to take drugs?

Good question! How do you answer this for the kid to whom you have fed mood-altering chemicals since he was in the third grade? As usual, the best approach is to do your homework ahead of time. Learn as much as you can about chemical health, and then teach it to your child. When faced with the challenge of comparing the risks of taking prescribed Dexedrine to smoking marijuana, for instance, perhaps a good place to start is with the law. A child already prone to high-risk behaviors might be more impressed with the threat of landing in jail than with a discussion of the health dangers of street drugs.

Drugs are a natural, lifelong issue for anyone with ADD. Many ADD teenagers turn to illegal drugs to self-medicate. They look to relieve the symptoms of their disorder, to settle down. And while they may feel stigmatized among their peers by taking a prescribed medication, especially if they're taking the same one they took as a small child, they often receive a different peer reaction to experimenting with illegal drugs. For someone who has been taking medications for most of his life, and who is reaching a rebellious stage, trying marijuana or cocaine is not a huge leap. But it can be a dangerous one.

One study of adults with ADHD reported that well over half have experienced substance abuse problems. People with ADHD also become addicted three times quicker than people without ADHD; they also take much longer to achieve remission, with more relapses. And it's no surprise that, by far, the greatest risk period is during the teenage years.

This is an age of exaggerated highs and lows, and there are no guarantees that your best efforts will ensure a trouble-free cruise through adolescence. But education and prevention are your best bet. Temper your efforts with enough patience to keep the lines of communication open. More than ever before, it's important to know what's going on in your kid's head, even as he struggles to become independent of you.

Parents need to watch for the signs of substance abuse in their children's rooms, in their behavior, and in their friends. Inevitably, this will lead to skirmishes over the issue of trust. When it does, we can tell our children that we trust them, but that we don't trust the disease of chemical dependency. During the rough ride through adolescence, there are times when it will become tempting to throw up your hands and give up. Remember that your constant love, support, and vigilance can make a crucial difference.

Hope for the Future

The proven existence of living ADD adults

It's one thing when a child can't stay on task well enough to get a home-work assignment done. But what about later, when this person faces the same problems on the job? A child acting out in an elementary school classroom might be disciplined or given a time-out. The child may be described as having ADD, perhaps even as oppositional and defiant. But what happens when an adult acts out at work or in public? The adult may be considered antisocial or dangerous.

The earlier we teach personal responsibility to our kids, the better off we all are. There's a fine line between having an awareness of a disability and using that disability as an excuse. Employers don't spend a lot of time considering an employee's psycho-educational assessment when dis-cipline problems arise on the job. The police and the courts don't either. The law offers no special exemptions for those who are distractible or have a hard time concentrating.

What is clear is that the skills we nurture in our children to get them through the day and the school year will need to last them through life. Eventually, we will probably not be around to reinforce them on a daily basis. Our children will go out into the world, enter into relationships, have car keys, handle their finances, be old enough to drink, and encounter the availability of other drugs. And they will still very likely have ADD.

The consistent love and discipline we offer now can reap rewards for our children later. We hope that they will be the foundation of our children's sense of self-esteem and that they will someday help buoy them through difficult times.

Through this maze of distraction, we must somehow keep our children's visions fixed on their dreams. We must remember that success or failure in school is not necessarily an indicator of success or failure in adult life. A dear friend of mine who works with challenged (and challenging) kids says: "Keep 'em alive till they're twenty-five." These words are now permanently emblazoned in my brain. There is just no way of knowing when someone's life will come into focus. We need to keep our kids safe and with some sense of self-esteem until that day arrives.

One of the best counselors we ever met was an ADHD adult. It took only a minute with him to see this: You could suffer whiplash just sitting in a room with him. After observing his energy level, organizational skills, and the condition of his office, you might guess he'd never gotten

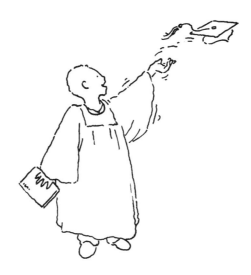

a handle on his disability. His doctorate degree, however, and, more important, the skills and professionalism he used while working with us showed he'd found a way.

We've all seen plenty of kids who struggled through their childhood and school years only to blossom later, becoming successful and happy adults. Kids with ADHD grow up to be artists, teachers, athletes, entrepreneurs, and doctors. These are kids who learned to gather up their lemons and use their incredible energy to make lemonade. These are kids who wouldn't give up on themselves, and they likely had parents who wouldn't give up either.

Through the shortcomings, frustrations, and failures, we cannot lose track of our children's heroic efforts. It takes resilience for them to withstand a world that chips away daily at their self-esteem, and to come back again the next day, full-speed ahead, with an energetic, caring, and joyfully sociable nature. So we must also keep our own visions fixed, maybe not on the dreams we started out with for our children, but on the life that we can help them build for themselves.

HELP!

Books, groups, and other resources

The conventional treatment for ADD is based on a combination of individual and family education and therapy, behavior management programs, and medication. Many people benefit from the medications used to treat ADD. However, some people have been frightened by the highly publicized controversy around the possible overprescription of Ritalin. Some need to try several different medications before they find one that works for them. Some are not helped by medication at all. As in any other part of your life, it's best to be an informed consumer.

There are alternative treatments for ADD as well, including some nutritionally based programs and some using vitamins and herbs. They seem to be based on common sense: controlling the intake of refined sugar and food additives. I am certainly not one to recommend one approach over another. From the perspective of a parent rather than a medical professional, it seems most reasonable to seek help from people you trust, listen to all points of view, and try what seems best until you find what works. You and your child will probably be the best judge of that.

There are many books available on ADD/ADHD, most of which are written by medical professionals. The following is a list of books that I have found to be informative. Each presents material in an appropriate manner for parents and family members who are not health care professionals. The organizations listed afterward are also sources of additional publications.

Barkley, Russell A., Ph.D. *Taking Charge of ADHD: The Complete, Authoritative Guide for Parents*. New York: Guilford Press, 1995.

Hallowell, Edward M., M.D., and John J. Ratey, M.D. *Driven to Distraction: Recognizing and Coping with Attention Deficit Disorder from Childhood through Adulthood*. New York: Simon and Schuster, 1995.

Hallowell, Edward M., M.D., and John J. Ratey, M.D. *Answers to Distraction*. New York: Bantam Books, 1996.

Kilcarr, Patrick J., Ph.D., and Patricia O. Quinn, M.D. *Voices from Fatherhood: Fathers, Sons and ADHD*. New York: Brunner/Mazel, 1997.

Silver, Larry, M.D. *Dr. Larry Silver's Advice to Parents on Attention-Deficit Hyperactivity*. Washington, D.C.: American Psychiatric Press, 1992.

Organizations that offer advocacy, support, and information for people with ADD, their parents, and their families include the following. These organizations may also be able to refer you to agencies or organizations within your community that can offer additional support.

Children and Adults with Attention Deficit Disorder (CHADD)
499 Northwest 70th Avenue
Suite 101
Plantation, FL 33317
(954) 587-3700
http://www.chadd.org

CHADD describes itself as the nation's leading organization working to improve the lives of people with ADD. Through family support and advocacy, public and professional education, and encouragement of scientific and educational research, CHADD works on behalf of children and adults with ADD. There are local chapters in every part of the United States. CHADD also publishes a newsletter, *Chadder Box,* and *Attention!* magazine.

iation (ADDA)

National Attention Deficit Disorder Association
Phone: (847) 432-ADDA

CHADD
Phone: (301) 306-7070

http://www.add.org

ADDA is an organization built around the needs of adults and young adults with ADD and ADHD. They seek to serve individuals with ADD, as well as those who love, live with, teach, counsel, and treat those who do.

About the Author

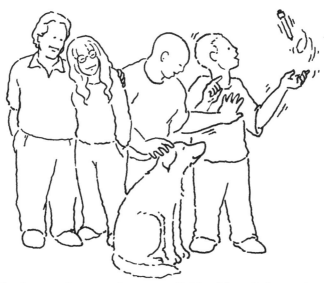

David Spohn is the art director of Hazelden Information and Educational Services, an author and illustrator of four children's books, and the father of a child with an attention deficit disorder. He lives in Lindstrom, Minnesota.

Hazelden Information and Educational Services is a division of the Hazelden Foundation, a not-for-profit organization. Since 1949, Hazelden has been a leader in promoting the dignity and treatment of people afflicted with the disease of chemical dependency.

The mission of the foundation is to improve the quality of life for individuals, families, and communities by providing a national continuum of information, education, and recovery services that are widely accessible; to advance the field through research and training; and to improve our quality and effectiveness through continuous improvement and innovation.

Stemming from that, the mission of this division is to provide quality information and support to people wherever they may be in their personal journey— from education and early intervention, through treatment and recovery, to personal and spiritual growth.

Although our treatment programs do not necessarily use everything Hazelden publishes, our bibliotherapeutic materials support our mission and the Twelve Step philosophy upon which it is based. We encourage your comments and feedback.

The headquarters of the Hazelden Foundation are in Center City, Minnesota. Additional treatment facilities are located in Chicago, Illinois; New York, New York; Plymouth, Minnesota; St. Paul, Minnesota; and West Palm Beach, Florida. At these sites, we provide a continuum of care for men and women of all ages. Our Plymouth facility is designed specifically for youth and families.

For more information on Hazelden, please call **1-800-257-7800.** Or you may access our World Wide Web site on the Internet at **http://www.hazelden.org.**